BOOK OF DOG NAMES

BOOK OF DOG NAMES

Simon Jeans

PENGUIN BOOKS

PENGUIN BOOKS

Published by the Penguin Group
Penguin Books Ltd, 27 Wrights Lane, London W8 5TZ, England
Penguin Books USA Inc., 375 Hudson Street, New York, New York 10014, USA
Penguin Books Australia Ltd, Ringwood, Victoria, Australia
Penguin Books Canada Ltd, 10 Alcorn Avenue, Toronto, Ontario,
Canada M4V 3B2
Penguin Books (NZ) Ltd, 182–190 Wairau Road, Auckland 10, New Zealand

Penguin Books Ltd, Registered Offices: Harmondsworth, Middlesex, England

First published in Australia by The Watermark Press 1992
Published in Penguin Books 1994
1 3 5 7 9 10 8 6 4 2

Cartoons reproduced by the kind permission of The New Yorker Magazine, Inc.

Additional drawings copyright © Sophie Blackall

Filmset in 10/12pt ITC Cheltenham Book by
Rowland Phototypesetting Ltd, Bury St Edmunds, Suffolk

Printed in England by Clays Ltd, St Ives plc

INTRODUCTION

What's in a name? More than most of us ever contemplate. Because a pet's name can be quirky, even eccentric, often more thought and research goes into the selection than that which is applied to the name of a child.

Here we provide examples from many sources and information on previous bearers of the name. There's Bud who walked from Mexico to Kansas in the best Lassie tradition. And, speaking of Lassie, her alter ego was Pal, a *laddie* who lived in luxury until he died at the age of nineteen.

In this small book are names of dogs both famous and obscure. Some are royal, many literary, a few cinematic, others historical, some musical.

Included are suggestions for different breeds, different colours, different personalities. There are names for guard dogs, lap dogs, family dogs and working dogs. Whatever your taste, you are sure to find a name befitting your pampered pet, one that will be a credit to you, both when you shout it aloud in public places or say it more quietly at home.

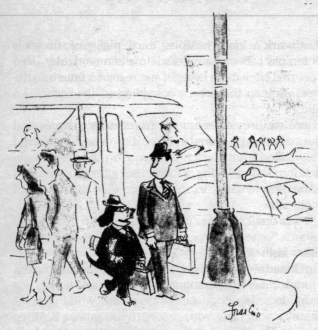

'I started out carrying his newspaper
and fetching his slippers. Then,
gradually, I began assuming more and
more responsibilities.'

Drawing by P. Frascino; © 1990 The New Yorker Magazine, Inc.

A

Aardvark Actually meaning 'earth pig', an aardvark is a cross between an armadillo and an anteater. This would be a good, original name for an unusual-looking, throwback sort of a dog.

Achilles Celebrated hero of Homer's epic the *Iliad*, known for his strength, energy and bravery. Heel, Achilles, heel!

Adah A good name for a female dog, as it means 'ornament' in Hebrew. Insist on the 'h', and give its pronunciation an aristocratic ring.

Adonis In classical Greek mythology Adonis was a beautiful youth, beloved of Aphrodite, killed by a boar while hunting. Not a name to take lightly.

Aglaia This is the name of one of the three Graces, meaning 'splendour', 'beauty'. It is rather doubtful whether you will ever meet another Aglaia, and you will enjoy explaining it.

Agnes *See* **Taggy**, **Talgert**.

Ahenobarbus This was the surname of a Roman family, of which the emperor Nero was the last member. It actually means 'yellow beard'. A perfect name for the hound with a long, shaggy goatee and a cowardly streak. *See* **Nero**.

Alard Meaning 'noble' and 'hard', this is a name with lofty connections.

Alfred Alfred means elf-counsel, elves being powerful nature spirits to the Anglo-Saxons. Or after the English king who failed in his role as assistant baker by allowing the cakes to burn – for a dog who has been known to cause minor domestic disasters!

Amanda From the Latin *amare*, Amanda means 'lovable'. The diminutive **Mandy** is more commonly used for dogs.

Ambrose From Greek mythology, meaning the fabled food and drink of the immortals, and hence the elixir of life. For the little pup who is the apple of your eye.

Ambleth, Amlet *See* **Hamlet**.

Angus This good Scottish name comes from the Gaelic, meaning 'unique choice' and has the very handy diminutive of **Gus**.

Anna *See* **Natasha**.

Annis *See* **Taggy**, **Talgert**.

Antony If your dog has changeable affections, name him after Marc Antony, who deserted his wife for the charms of **Cleopatra**.

Argos Odysseus returned home in diguise after a twenty-year absence, as he still feared for his life. The only one who recognized him was his little dog Argos, who died of joy when he saw his master.

Arthur This popular name originates from Celtic words connected with 'bear' and became popular due to the fame of King Arthur of the Round Table.

Ascot One of the highlights of the British racing calendar where racegoers dress to impress and the champagne flows. A good name for a dog who enjoys the big occasion.

Asta The pet of Nick and Nora Charles, of the *Thin Man* films.

Asterix A cult comic-book hero, Goscinny's and Uderzo's tiny Gaul lives in a village in northern France and keeps the Romans at bay with the help of his dull-minded friend, Obelix, and Getafix the druid's magic potion. *See* **Dogmatix**, **Obelix**.

Astro The lazy but lovable dog in the space-age cartoon series *The Jetsons*. This name would suit larger breeds such as Great Danes or Irish Wolfhounds.

Attila King of the Huns, called the 'Scourge of God'. Attila ravaged the Roman Empire before suffering his only defeat at Châlons-sur-Marne. For the dog who likes to mark his territory.

Aubrey This is a good name for shorter breeds, deriving from the Old German name Alberic, king of the dwarfs. Oberon, the elfin king in Shakespeare's *A Midsummer Night's Dream*, is another name derived from Alberic.

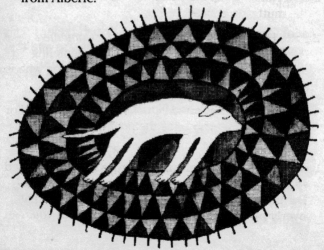

B

Bacall If you wonder what you've ever done to deserve your dog, name her after the beautiful screen actress Lauren Bacall.

Bacchus *See* **Denis, Dennis**.

Bagel For a dog who enjoys a wholesome roll.

Bailey The dog who roams may be named for 'Won't you come home?' Bill Bailey.

Baloo Rudyard Kipling's bear in *The Jungle Book*. For the mutt with a sweet tooth.

Balzac Honoré de Balzac, author of *La Comédie Humaine*, a work of over fifty volumes depicting aspects of contemporary society. For the dog who is a good judge of character.

Bandit or **Bandito**, meaning a lawless desperado. For the outlaw dog who bites the postman and chases the milkman.

Barnum Phineas T. Barnum, of circus fame, is claimed to have said, 'There's a sucker born every minute.' For the dog who could be in the circus or for that overly pampered pooch making a sucker of *you*.

Barry Barry was the name of a courageous St Bernard who rescued at least forty travellers lost in the snowy Alps between Switzerland and Italy at the turn of the eighteenth century.

Basil From the Greek, meaning 'kingly'. But if your pooch does not live up to such a regal moniker, just think instead of John Cleese's neurotic Basil Fawlty in *Fawlty Towers*.

Beatrice *See* **Trixie**.

Beaumont Ben Jonson wrote of fellow playwright Francis Beaumont that 'he loved too much himself and his own verse.' So if your dog is an egotist, Beaumont would be ideal.

Beecher 'The dog was created specifically for children. He is the god of frolic.' So wrote Henry Ward Beecher in *Proverbs from Plymouth Pulpit* (1887).

Bell There are so many derivations that we can only give a few. It may be an abbreviation of Isabel; or of Bellerophon, who attempted to fly to heaven on Pegasus; or of Bellona, the Roman goddess of war.

Bella, Belle In Italian and French 'lovely' and 'beautiful', Bella is probably more commonly used than Belle.

Benedictine An order of monks who were renowned for their learning and played an influential part in the civilization of Europe. For the sober and serious hound.

Benji Benji, a modern shortening of the ancient Hebrew name Benjamin, 'son of the right hand', is a very popular dog's name. Probably more so since the film *For the Love of Benji*.

Bentley If you dog likes to travel in style, why not name him after one of the all-time classic cars, whose elegance and performance were motoring perfection? Other similar names could be **Roller**, **Daimler** or **Jaguar**. Or, if he's a speed-hound, **Lotus** or **Maclaren**.

Beowulf This eighth-century poem tells of a courageous Geatish hero who defeats a hideous monster only to be ultimately slain by a dragon. Perfect for a vigilant guard dog.

Bernard The St Bernard dog of Switzerland was named after St Bernard of Menthon who founded the alpine hospice for travellers. Some common short forms are Bernie, Barney and Nardie. *See* **Barry**.

Bert A good short name for a dog with loads of personality. Or for one half of a duo with **Ernie** after the *Sesame Street* characters.

Bertha A goddess of German ancestry, sometimes prefaced with Big. For the larger females.

Bevis In Sir Walter Scott's poem 'Marmion' Bevis was the name of the red-roan charger. Bevis was also one of King Arthur's knights. It is a name suggesting chivalry and a shiny red coat.

Blackie An affectionate family name but highly unoriginal for a black pooch.

Blondel According to popular legend, Blondel was a young troubadour who wandered Bohemia in search of Richard the Lionheart, singing a coded song until his imprisoned king responded. For the dog who howls when there's a full moon.

Boatswain Byron was a great animal lover, and had a small menagerie in his house in Italy, including his enormous and much beloved black Newfoundland Boatswain (pronounced Bosun). The unfortunate dog died of rabies.

Bobby After Greyfriars Bobby who waited patiently for his dead master. There's a statue to his memory in Edinburgh.

Bogarde/Bogart Dirk or Humphrey. For dogs who talk tough but have a heart of gold underneath.

Bond James Bond, 007, the creation of Ian Fleming. Would suit a suave male dog popular with the ladies who likes his doggy drinks shaken, not stirred. Grrrrr!

Bonzo A humorous dog created by George Studdy in 1912. Bonzo enjoyed popularity for many years; his image was reproduced on postcards, toys and in films. A light-hearted and comical name.

Boo Boo Yogi Bear's companion. For the little pup who makes a few mistakes.

Boogaloo For that frolicsome, dancing dog.

Boogie Boogie-woogie was a style of piano playing cultivated by early twentieth-century jazz musicians. You and your canine would have to possess incredible talent or 'boogie fever' to live up to this name.

Boris This name derives from a Russian word meaning 'fight'. For aggressive dogs of Russian descent. It also calls to mind the battling and athletic tennis star Boris Becker, famous for his leaps across the court, which occasionally landed him on the deck.

Boswell James Boswell, politician and author of *The Life of Samuel Johnson* (1791), was described after the discovery of his papers in the 1920s as the 'best self-documented man in all history'. For the dog who faithfully takes note of everything.

Bounce The poet Alexander Pope, who was very frail and seriously handicapped, had a protector in his Great Dane, Bounce. The huge hound actually saved Pope from an attack by a corrupt servant.

Bounder For that irrepressible cur that cuts a great caper.

Bows *See* **Buttons**.

Bowser Derived from 'drunkard', this would suit a lively dog who likes a regular bottle of milk.

Boy The earliest Poodle heard of in Britain, Boy was given to Prince Rupert of the royal Stuarts during his imprisonment at Linz in 1640. The pooch was feared by Cromwellian soldiers, who thought he was a dog-witch with the gift of languages and prophecy.

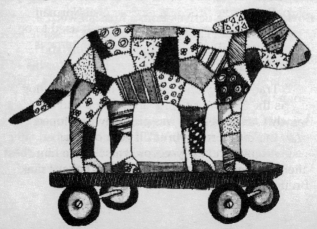

Brag There is an old saying, 'Brag is a good dog, but Holdfast is better,' which means that doing something is better than just talking about it. Shakespeare alludes to it in *Henry V*:

Trust none;
For oaths are straws, men's faiths are wafer-cakes,
And hold-fast is the only dog, my duck.

So Brag for a dog who barks but never bites?

Bran The dog of Fingal, the legendary Irish hero, was a great favourite and is mentioned in Scott's *Waverley*: 'If not Bran, then it is Bran's brother' (in every way as good).

Bruce Deriving no doubt from the thirteenth-century hero, Robert the Bruce. The name is of Norman origin, and Brewis is one of its forms. It used to be enormously popular, but nowadays the name is considered a tad ordinary.

Bruno Traditionally, this is a name for a brown dog. It was the name of an early archbishop and a saintly Carthusian and was probably developed from the Old German 'brun'. If your dog has championship hopes, you could also name him after the popular British heavyweight boxer Frank Bruno.

Brutus This Roman suffered agonies of mind when he became embroiled in the plot to stab Julius Caesar to death. For the hound who brings his daggers out when your back is turned.

Buck The canine hero of Jack London's classic tale of survival in a husky pack in the frozen north, *Call of the Wild*. It also brings to mind the hero from the TV series *Buck Rogers in the Twenty-Fifth Century*.

Buckingham If your dog has a dandified air and thoroughly enjoys being on show, this name suggests one of the dashing beaux of the English Regency period.

Bud In the tradition of *Lassie Come Home*, a collie named Bud travelled 800 miles to rejoin his departed American owners when they moved. A good name for a faithful dog.

Bumble Reminiscent of the bee and so a perfect name for a barrel-shaped brindle dog. Also the name of the beadle in Dickens's *Oliver Twist*, who brings us the term 'bumbledom', meaning 'foolish officiousness'.

Bummer If your pooch scrounges through dustbins, or if he's just footloose, here's a good name.

Buster A vulgar form of 'burster', implying an abundance of vitality or something that takes one's breath away. Also an affectionate term akin to 'buddy'.

Butch Outlaws Butch Cassidy and the Sundance Kid occupy a favourable place in popular history, due mainly to the Hollywood film starring Paul Newman and Robert Redford.

Butterscotch A cheerful name for a dog with a caramel-coloured coat – say, a Golden Labrador.

Buttons Bright as a button: well suited to a lively and playful pup. Or for a pup with a wistful air, name him after the lovelorn kitchen boy in the traditional pantomime of Cinderella. If you have a pair of cute little dogs, who couldn't possibly survive without their regular shampoo and delicate foods, why not name them **Buttons** and **Bows**?

C

Caesar A Wire-haired Terrier named Caesar was the last and best-loved dog of King Edward VII. He once bit the seat of the then Prime Minister, Herbert Asquith, who sat in the mutt's chair by mistake. The titles Kaiser and Tsar are variants of the name.

Camelot A name redolent of Arthurian legend. Whether it or its king existed or not, the name conjures up the adventure and chivalry of the Round Table. A name for a fearless dog who always seems to be on a quest for new adventures.

Camp Sir Walter Scott's devotion to dogs is evident in his books. Camp was a crossbreed, part Bulldog, part Rat Terrier.

Campbell The name of a noble Scottish clan. This would be a perfect name for a West Highland White or a Scottish Terrier.

Candy A sweet name. No need to worry about this dog's bite; its teeth should be completely rotten.

Caper For the bouncy hound who likes to jump about.

Capulet A noble name, taken from one of the feuding families in Shakespeare's *Romeo and Juliet*. Juliet came from the Capulets and Romeo from the Montagues. If your pooch is having an ongoing conflict with a dog down the road, then this would fit the bill.

Carmen After the tragic heroine of Bizet's famous opera. For a dog who loves drama and to be centre-stage.

Cassidy *See* **Butch**.

Cato This spaniel was a gift from Henry VII to his ambassador Lord Wiltshire, who took him on a diplomatic visit to the Pope in Rome. In an age-old gesture the Pope extended his toe to the Lord, but Cato misunderstood, bit the papal toe and was hacked to death by the papal guards.

Cavall King Arthur of Round Table fame's favourite dog.

Cerberus *See* **Pluto**.

Charles The names of three Merovingian kings of France will amuse: Charles the Bald (823–877), Charles the Fat (839–888) and Charles the Simple (879–929). Take your choice.

Charley Author John Steinbeck travelled America with his dog Charley and later wrote a book about their adventures, appropriately titled *Travels with Charley*.

Chester A historic English town where some of the mystery plays were performed. It still retains many of its characterful old streets and buildings.

Chico *See* **Groucho**.

Chip One half of the chipmunk duo Chip and **Dale**, from the Walt Disney cartoon. Ideal for a small, mischievous dog.

Cicero From the Latin word 'cicer', meaning wart. Marcus Tullius, the great Roman statesman, was called Cicero because he had a small growth on the top of his nose. May be abbreviated to Cissy.

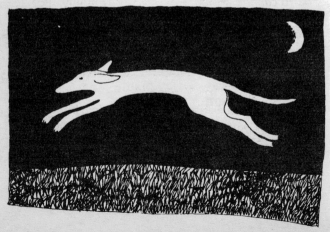

Claude Comes from a clan name probably meaning 'limping'. When Claudius became Roman emperor, many flattered him by asserting his name came from a word meaning 'glorious'. For the dog who hears only what it wants to.

Cleopatra Name a queenly dog after the beautiful African queen of Egypt, who devastated the Roman general Marc **Antony** with her beauty. For a dog that casts a spell on all who see her.

Clint From Clint 'Go ahead, make my day' Eastwood.

Coco Choose this name for a dog, and it may live up to Chanel's reputation for simple, yet elegant, lines.

Colin Colin, though it may not sound like it, is the perfect name for a dog. It derives from the Celtic word *cailean*, which means 'a young hound'. It is possible that the name Collie also derives from this word.

Colonel A name used in *101 Dalmatians* by Dodie Smith. Other regimental titles can also be suitable for the right character. *See* **Major**.

Conrad Sometimes used for a roving dog, but it is also apt for an analytical dog, following in the footsteps of the writer Joseph Conrad (1857–1924).

Cornflakes For a dog that's a bit flaky but very much part of the family. A fun name for a children's pet.

Crusoe A good name for a dog thrown back on its own resources – perhaps for a stray who learns to adapt to a new life.

Cuchulain Name an Irish Wolfhound after this great Irish hero, known as the Hound of Ulster.

Cupid Charles II was a great dog lover (King Charles Spaniels are named for him). The first Spaniel he owned was given to him after his coronation and was named Cupid. For the dog who steals your heart.

D

Daimler *See* **Bentley**.

Daisy This name actually derives from the Anglo-Saxon 'day's eye' because the daisy closes its petals as night approaches. For the pooch who appears fresh as a daisy in the morning.

Dale *See* **Chip**.

Dandy Associations span from the Dandie Dinmont breed of terriers to an elegantly dressed fop.

Danny The abbreviated form of the biblical name Daniel also has associations with Irish folk music ('Oh, Danny Boy') and movie star (Danny Kaye). For the multi-talented mutt.

Dante The name itself is an abbreviation of Durante, which comes from the Latin 'lasting'.

Darwin What more inspiring name could you give to a dog than that of Charles Darwin, the man who gave us the modern theory of evolution? To paraphrase Darwin, it's survival of the fittest in this dog-eat-dog world.

Dash In pidgin English, dash can mean a free gift, so if your family pet was given to you as a present, then this could fit. It is also a euphemism for 'damn', used in the nineteenth century as an inoffensive swear word.

Deimos The planet **Mars** has two satellites, Deimos and **Phobos**, words from the Greek meaning 'panic' and 'terror'. They are very close to the planet and difficult to observe from Earth. Appropriate for an inseparable duo or trio.

Delilah That beautiful but treacherous woman of 'Samson and Delilah' fame (Judges: XVI). See **Samson**.

Denis, Dennis This name derives from the Greek Dionysus, better known as Bacchus. Dennis is the Irish version, and the name of a popular comic character, Dennis the Menace, who lives up to his name. For the mischievous pup who digs up your roses or chews your slippers.

Devil For your own little devil, either a large, fierce-looking dog or, ironically, a small, harmless terrier.

Diamond Diamond, the little dog of Sir Isaac Newton, the famous seventeenth-century scientist and astronomer, once set fire to records of experiments Newton was working on by accidentally knocking over a candle. For the clumsy but lovable mutt.

Diggory From the French *égaré*, 'strayed' or 'lost', this is a very good name should your dog happen to be a foundling. Thomas Hardy used it for a character in *The Return of the Native* (Diggory Venn), C.S. Lewis named one of the children in the Narnia Chronicles Diggory, and it was also the name of the rustic serving man in *She Stoops to Conquer* by Oliver Goldsmith.

Dino For the dog that bowls you over when you walk in the door and then eagerly licks your face. All you can say is 'Down, boy,' as does Fred Flintstone in the TV cartoon *The Flintstones*.

Disney Walt Disney (1901–1966), the great cartoon film producer and creator of Mickey Mouse, Donald Duck, *et al.*

Dog When nothing else seems to fit. And, as Aldous Huxley pointed out in *Antic Hay*, it spells 'God' backwards.

Dogmatix Asterix's small, white, Gaulish dog from the Asterix comic strip series. *See* **Asterix**, **Obelix**.

Domini Canes Literally, 'Hounds of the Lord', this name was applied to the order founded by the Spaniard St Dominic. To make it easier to call out, it can be abbreviated to Dom.

Domino An ideal name for a Dalmatian or in praise of Fats Domino, the musician.

Dookie *See* **Windsor**.

Dorothy Dorothy derives from the Greek words *doron*, meaning 'gift', and *theou*, meaning 'of God'. It brings to mind Dorothy from the classic *The Wizard of Oz*. Shortenings include Dot, Dottie, Dodo, Dodie and Dora.

Dougal Dougal the dog, star of the BBC children's television series *The Magic Roundabout*, elevated the series to cult status with his cynical quips. For a dog with a woldly-wise, or world-weary air.

Duchess Like Princess, **Prince, King** and Queenie, this is a highly unoriginal name, but small children love it.

Dudley One of a number of illustrious surnames, most belonging to ancient, noble families. Gradually they have come into use as first names. If your dog is small but perfectly formed, name him after the musician and comedy star of the *Arthur* films, Dudley Moore.

Duke Derived from *dux*, meaning 'leader' in Latin, whence came the title 'Il Duce' for Benito Mussolini, the Italian Fascist dictator. It was also Hollywood Western star John Wayne's nickname, which he took from a childhood pet.

Dylan For either Bob Dylan or Dylan Thomas. If your
pup seems to be a budding poet or sings a bit off-
key, this may be the perfect name.

E

E.T. Steven Spielberg's immortal character E.T. was not the most handsome of creatures, so bear that in mind when you name the odd-looking beast that arrived on your doorstep, seemingly out of nowhere.

Einstein Possibly a good name for a slow starter. Albert Einstein's parents feared he was backward during his early school years. Then in 1916 he produced his revolutionary general theory of relativity.

Elsa Most famous as the lioness in the book *Born Free*, Elsa could also apply to dogs of the more leonine breeds such as Collies or German Shepherds.

Elvis Presley, the King. A perfect name for a hound dog.

Engels The German political figure Friedrich Engels wrote *The Condition of the Working Class in England* in 1844, co-wrote *The Communist Manifesto* with Marx in 1848 and completed *Das Kapital* in 1894 after Marx died. Strictly for the working-class mutt.

Erasmus Desiderius Erasmus (*c.* 1466–1536), the Dutch Renaissance theologian and scholar.

Erin An ancient and poetic name for Ireland, perfect for an Irish Wolfhound.

Ernest The importance of being earnest – this name means what it says. Short forms are Ern and Ernie. Think of naming a pair Bert and Ernie after the quarrelsome duo in *Sesame Street*.

Errol Hollywood's great swashbuckler and charming rogue of the late 1930s and early 1940s, Errol Flynn starred in such films as *Captain Blood* and *The Adventures of Robin Hood*. Only for a dog who steals bones from the rich to give to the poor.

Erebus In Greek mythology Erebus was the son of Chaos and the brother of Night. Darkness personified. For the coal-black dog.

F

Faith A fine name for the dog who was sold to you as a pedigreed pooch, but whose breeder somehow just couldn't find the registration papers. It also suggests the loyalty and faithfulness of man's best friend.

Falstaff A great name for a big Old English Sheepdog, named after one of Shakespeare's greatest characters, the wily and rumbustious mentor of Prince Hal in *Henry IV* and *Henry V*.

Faramund Although of German origin, this name was brought to England by the Normans. It is a compound of *fara*, meaning 'journey', and *mund*, meaning 'protection'. Good for a traveller's dog.

Farquhar The name of an early eighteenth-century Irish playwright.

Fatty One of the puppies in *101 Dalmatians* by Dodie Smith. Also brings to mind entertainers Fatty Arbuckle and Fats Domino.

Felix Although from the legendary cartoon cat of the same name, it can still be applied to a cheerful, friendly dog, as Felix means 'lucky', 'happy'. *See also* **Oscar**.

Ferdinand Same derivation as **Faramund**. For the adventurous dog who has maybe watched *Lassie Come Home* one too many times.

Fergus 'Manly choice' or 'supreme choice', it was a popular name for Celtic saints. Fergus is still common in Scotland, as is the surname Ferguson. Gus would be stretching it.

Fido This name comes from the Latin *fidelio* meaning 'the faithful one'. It has become *the* generic dog name.

Fifi The shortened form of Fiona should only be used for that very small, very pampered French poodle.

Flora Flora Macdonald helped the fugitive Bonnie Prince Charlie to escape to Skye, by disguising him as her maidservant. A good name for a loyal and resourceful dog.

Floss This is, of course, an abbreviation of Florence, rarely used before the fame of Florence Nightingale, the 'Lady with the Lamp', gave it fresh impetus. It is a homely name that needs no apology.

Flush Elizabeth Barrett's spaniel, Flush, was nearly destroyed by the poet's father after her romantic elopement with Robert Browning. Her sister and a servant managed to sneak Flush out of the home, and he lived with Barrett to the end of his days.

Flynn *See* **Errol**.

Franco This Spanish dictator was not renowned for his benign policies on human rights, so your dog might use this name as a cue for antisocial behaviour.

Franklin A dog named Franklin is the perfect companion when flying a kite in a thunderstorm – which, of course, was how Benjamin Franklin discovered electricity.

Franz A dog can sometimes feel he is in an enigmatic and callous world, riddled with guilt and loneliness, where the ordinary often becomes sinister. The Czech novelist Franz Kafka wrote about such feelings, so let your dog know he's not alone out there.

Freckles Ideal for a dog with a pied or ticked coat, perhaps a Dalmatian or a German Short-haired Pointer.

Fred Is your dog as light on his feet as Fred Astaire or companion to another pet named Ginger? Either way, this is a simple and pleasant name. If you have a Bassett hound, it's going to be hard to avoid this choice of name, after the famous canine character Fred Bassett.

Freddy/Freddie Freddy is actually an old German compound of *frithu*, which means 'peace', and *ric*, which means 'ruler'. If your hound has unusually long claws, name him after *Nightmare on Elm Street* baddie Freddie Krueger.

Friday In Defoe's novel Crusoe's companion was Man Friday – but why not Dog Friday or, indeed, any other day of the week?

Fritz Would suit a Germanic breed, in particular the Dachshund.

Frodo Noted character from J.R.R. Tolkien's magical fantasy novels. A wonderful name for a woodsy type of dog with a sense of humour.

Fungus Raymond Briggs's *Fungus the Bogeyman* is a picture book that has enjoyed cult status. The subterranean life-style of the Bogeys and their dislike of the 'Dry Cleaners', or humans, has repelled and delighted adults and children alike.

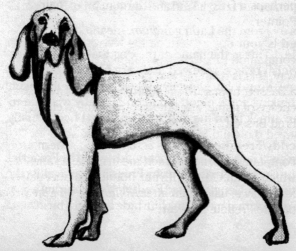

G

Gable *See* **King**.

Galileo Galileo Galilei (1564–1642), the Italian astronomer, established the scientific testing of theories and was among the first to use a telescope for astronomy. Only for the star-struck dog.

Garnet For a precious dog, as a garnet is a jewel.

Gatsby For a dog who loves to put on the Ritz, this name evokes the sultry mood of the Twenties and Scott Fitzgerald's novel, a tale of passion set among the glamour of Long Island and the squalor of New York.

Gaudy From the Latin *gaudium*, meaning joy.

Gelert This is the name of the dog that Llewellyn, a Welsh prince, received in dowry from his father-in-law, King John. Llewellyn killed him after mistakenly thinking some blood found on his baby was due to an attack from the dog. Instead Gelert had actually saved the child from being killed by a wolf.

Gengist Gengist was a giant hound owned by Frederick the Great of Prussia. During Prussia's war against the Russians, Gengist saved Frederick's life during a Cossack raid by making him hide behind a bush.

George Virgil called his poems on farming the *Georgics* because George actually means 'tiller of the ground'. The most famous George was St George, patron saint of England, who killed a dragon. His day is 23 April. *See* **Virgil.**

Geronimo The Chiricahua Apache chief (1829–1909). 'Geronimo!' is also well known as the cry uttered before parachuting out of a plane. For the dog with a head for heights.

Gertrude The original Gertrude was one of the Valkyries, the maidens in Norse mythology who took those heroes killed on the battlefield to the palace of bliss, Valhalla. The name actually means 'spear-strength'.

Gilbert Together with Sir Arthur **Sullivan**, W.S. Gilbert created some of the all-time great comic operettas, such as *HMS Pinafore* and *The Pirates of Penzance*. However, they quarrelled during the run of *The Gondoliers*, supposedly over a new carpet at the Savoy Theatre in London, and did not speak to one another thereafter. For a pair of dogs with a tempestuous relationship.

Ginger From Middle English *gingivere*, this name denotes a redhead. A red Silky Terrier, perhaps.

Godzilla The name that applies to that ferocious screen monster, twice as big as the tallest skyscraper, could be quirkily applied to a little canine with a big bark.

Goethe Johann Wolfgang von Goethe wrote, 'Wanted: a dog that neither barks nor bites, eats broken glass and shits diamonds.'

Goldie Along with Wolf and **Prince**, Goldie was one of Hitler's German Shepherd dogs. Still, a pleasant enough name.

Goofy The name of this popular Disney dog, a friend of Mickey Mouse, has become synonymous with clumsiness.

Grenville *See* **Dudley**.

Grieg The name of Paul Newman's dog. Grieg, the Norwegian composer, is one of Newman's favourites.

Groke *See* **Moomin**.

Groucho One of the three Marx brothers, along with **Harpo** and Chico. The team originally included brothers Gummo and Zeppo. All extremely becoming dog names.

Growly A puppy in *101 Dalmatians* who aspired to be fierce.

Guinness Stout made by the firm of Guinness from Dublin. It is a rich and creamy black beer and so could refer to a dog of similar colouring.

Gus *See* **Angus**.

Gypsy Charles Dickens, himself a dog lover, introduced several dogs into his novels. A memorable one was the little spaniel Gypsy, always called Jip, who belonged to Dora, David Copperfield's 'child bride'.

H

Hamlet The only name for a mutt that has problems making up his mind or is overly fond of his mother. More archaic forms of the name are Amlet and Ambleth.

Happy The name of George V's royal dog. Also the name of one of the dwarfs in the 1937 Walt Disney cartoon *Snow White and the Seven Dwarfs*, appropriate if your pet is pint-sized.

Hardy See **Laurel**.

Harold See **Herald**.

Harpo Marx, the quiet one. See **Groucho**.

Harry Harry is a diminutive of Henry, which came about in an effort to imitate the French pronunciation of Henri. Hank is an American version.

Heathcliff The dark, powerful hero of Emily Brontë's *Wuthering Heights*. Always associated with darkness, it might suit a black dog. An impressive and potent name.

Hector The hero of Troy, slain by **Achilles**. A good name for a mean-looking dog that is always ready for a good fight.

Helen The Trojan War was her fault. Name your dog for this seductress, and you might find an invasion force at your doorstep.

Herald This, together with Heral, Herolt and several others, was an eleventh-century version of Harold. This could be the perfect name for the mutt who likes to fetch his owner's newspaper in the morning.

Holdfast *See* **Brag.**

Holmes The famous detective of Baker Street was known for his diligence when on the trail, as symbolized by his trademark deerstalker hat. For a dog with an insatiable curiosity, and a keen nose. *See also* **Watson**.

Homer The Greek epic poet. A fine name for the dog of heroic adventures.

Honey For the lovable light-coloured dog.

Horatio The faithful companion of **Hamlet** makes a delightful name for a canine friend.

Hosanna We are more likely to hear this as an exclamation at a revivalist meeting than to find that a friend has chosen it as a name for a dog. Still, a joyous name that deserves resurrection.

Hotei This is a Japanese name that is easy to pronounce (Ho-tay). In Japanese folklore, there were seven gods of luck; among them Hotei was the god of joviality.

Hotspur Shakespeare's Hotspur's real name was Sir Henry Percy, but he was better known as **Harry** Hotspur, a name which probably came from the impetuousness of his attacks.

Howard Howard Hughes, the fabulously rich recluse. A fine name for the dog who loves his little corner and won't leave it. *See* **Dudley**.

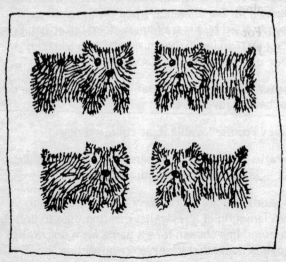

Huckleberry A rather cumbersome but charming name for an adventurous young dog. Easily shortened to Huck.

Hugo Victor Hugo (1802–1885), author and politician, apostle of Romanticism, libertarian, humanitarian and democratic idealist, who wrote *Les Misérables*. For an old and intelligent breed.

Humphrey There are several versions of this name, which was widely used in the Middle Ages. The original form was Humfrey. The nursery hero Humpty Dumpty was no doubt originally called Humfrey.

Hyde For the dog who has a good and a bad side. *See* **Jekyll**.

I

Isengrin *See* **Reynard**.

It Girl The name given to US film star Clara Bow, the sex goddess of Hollywood in the Roaring Twenties, reputed to have made love to an entire football team.

Ivan The Russian version of the name John. Ivan the Terrible, the first tsar of Russia, was a man of great cruelty. 'Ivan Ivanovitch' is used to denote the national personification of Russia, like the English 'John Bull'.

Ivor From a Welsh word meaning 'lord'. For the canine with royal lineage.

J

Jack The Scottish form of the name is **Jock**. Jack is a nickname for John; it became very common during the fourteenth-century – hence its wide use in nursery rhymes. There is Jack Horner, Jack and the Beanstalk and Jack and Jill, to name just a few. *See also* **Jake**.

Jackson There have been many famous Jacksons, from the steely Thomas 'Stonewall' Jackson, an American Confederate general, to the elfin, eccentric megastar Michael Jackson. So this name could be used for either a fearless conqueror or a dog with reclusive traits.

Jagger Name your dog after Mick Jagger if he's a rocker with great staying power.

Jake An American alternative to **Jack** or Jacques, which are nicknames for John.

Jason Of Golden Fleece fame. Or that twentieth-century golden boy, Jason Donovan, at one time star of the Australian soap opera *Neighbours* and now a successful pop singer and musical actor.

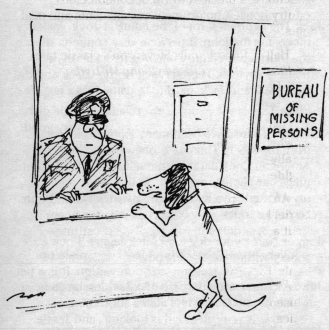

'He's about five feet six, has big brown
eyes and curly blond hair, and
answers to the name of Master.'

Drawing by Ross; © 1990 The New Yorker Magazine, Inc.

Jeeves This name, and that of **Wooster**, light-hearted names will evoke the japes and scrapes of P.G. Wodehouse's timeless world of London clubs, country houses, unfortunate engagements and mad aunts.

Jekyll Half of Robert Louis Stevenson's classic tale *The Strange Case of Dr Jekyll and Mr Hyde*, published in 1886.

Jemima This is the name of the rebellious little girl who, when she was good, could be very, very good, but when she was bad, she was horrid. The name actually means 'dove', and she was one of the daughters of Job.

Jenny An attractive and domestic name, which Dante Gabriel Rossetti used as the basis for his poem about a beautiful and flaxen-haired prostitute.

Jess A very popular name for a farm dog, male or female. In both cases it is an abbreviation. It is a pet name for any male dog called Jesse, Jessop (a form of Joseph) or Joshua. It is also a shortening of Jessica, which means 'God is looking', and Jessie.

Jester Why not give the cheerful clown in your house this name?

Jet Denoting a deep, glossy black dog, this name would suit a Labrador.

Jip *See* **Gypsy**.

Jock The feisty Scottish Terrier in that timeless Walt Disney film *Lady and the Tramp*.

Joplin Janis, the Sixties blues singer who was just as well known for her 'sex, drugs and rock'n'roll' lifestyle. An outrageously raunchy name, so make sure your dog can live up to it.

Joseph *See* **Jess**.

Josh Shortened form of Joshua. *See* **Jess**.

Jupiter The largest of the planets in the solar system, Jupiter is a Latin word corresponding to the Sanskrit for 'heavenly father'. Jupiter was also the supreme deity of the ancient Romans.

K

Katie, Katy An abbreviation of Katherine and the heroine of the celebrated children's novels by Susan Coolidge. For a small, cute dog.

Keeper Emily Brontë was a severe disciplinarian who frequently used the whip. Her Great Dane, Keeper, never left her side and was with her when she died.

Killer This name is not often bestowed seriously but rather in jest. Perfect for the dog who leads burglars to the family silver and runs from the neighbourhood cat.

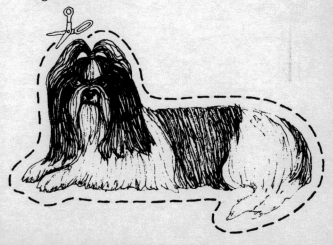

King Among its other numerous applications, the King was the nickname of Clark Gable, the much adored film star. Perfect for the mutt that has a way with the ladies.

King Kong The monster-size gorilla in the 1933 film that made the Empire State Building look small. Use this name for a burly Boxer with brawn.

L

La Fayette Marie-Madeleine Pioche de la Vergne, Comtesse de La Fayette, wrote *La Princesse de Clèves* (1678), a novel about a woman whose marriage is shattered by a guilty passion. A great name for a dainty dog, with the diminutive, Faye.

Ladon While hunting with his hounds, Actaeon unwittingly intruded upon Diana bathing in a pool. The goddess changed him into a stag and he was torn to pieces by his own hounds, one of them Ladon. There must be a dog for whom this name would be suitable.

Lady This is number one on *The Guinness Book of Names* list of the most popular names for dogs in the United States. There are many associations with this name: *Lady and the Tramp,* Lady Day, lady-in-waiting, ladykiller and Lady Luck.

Laelaps This would be an excellent name for a gun dog. In the legend of Procris and Cephalus, Procris fled from Cephalus and was aided by the goddess Diana, who gave her a dog, Laelaps, which never failed to secure its prey.

Laika The little Russian dog that became the first animal to be launched into orbit around the Earth during the space race between America and the USSR in the late 1950s and early 1960s.

Lalage This is a name used in a poem by Horace for a young girl, presumably a chatterbox, as the word means 'babbling'. For the dog that barks incessantly.

Lancelot Sir Lancelot, Knight of the Round Table and lover of King Arthur's wife Guinevere. For the dashing hound.

Lassie This name was made popular by a series of films about a Collie of exceptional qualities. Apparently the role was played by several different dogs, both male and female, over a period of two decades. *See* **Pal**.

Laurel Stanley Laurel and Oliver **Hardy**, an English and an American comedian respectively, together made one of cinema's greatest comedy acts. They won an Oscar in 1932 for *The Music Box*.

Lazarus This mongrel mutt, owned by the eccentric Emperor Norton I of America, had the biggest funeral for a dog on record in 1862. It was held in San Francisco and about 10,000 people attended.

Leary Timothy Leary, the advocate of LSD. A name that would suit a dog who tunes out, turns over and then drops off to sleep.

Leo The lion, from which names of heroes, saints and kings derive. The following lordly names originate from Leo: Leofric, Leofwin, Leon, Leonard, Leopold, Lionel and Lyall.

Lightning 'Thunder is good, thunder is impressive; but it is the lightning that does the work,' said Mark Twain. For the speedy hound with lots of energy.

Liline Liline was a favourite spaniel of Henry III of France, who had a superstitious faith in the judgement of these dogs. He once ignored her dislike of a visitor, Jacques Clement, who turned out to be his assassin.

Lionel *See* **Leo**.

Liquorice An appropriate name for a jet-black dog, maybe one who's always up to all sorts of pranks.

Lloyd Lloyd George, Britain's Prime Minister in the First World War. A sombre name.

Lotus *See* **Bentley**.

Lovell/Lovel A name from the Middle Ages, best remembered by the famous lines nailed to the door of St Paul's Cathedral in London in 1484:

> The cat, the rat, and Lovel our dog
> Rule all England under the hog.

Luath This was the name of the favourite dog of the Scottish poet Robert Burns. Irish mythology also has it that Luath was the name of a watchdog accidentally slain by the hero **Cuchulain**, who had to take the dog's place in penance.

Lucia, Lucy Names linked with virtuous persons, derived from *lux*, the Latin for light, these would be suitable for gentle creatures of pedigreed stock. Other derivations include Lucian, Lucius, Lucas, Lucille, Lucilla and Luke.

Lucifer This name, with its dual connotations of good and evil, should not be a casual choice. Milton's Lucifer was princely. One can visualize a proud, elegant creature, a superb guard dog.

Lucky For that fortuitous dog that will charm the household.

Ludwig Ludwig van Beethoven. For the dog who howls to 'Moonlight Sonata'.

Luke *See* **Lucia, Lucy**.

Lulu If you've got a bouncy little dog that's a real lulu, name her after the diminutive Scottish songstress who shot to fame in 1964 with her hit song 'Shout!'

Lupus Latin for 'wolf'.

Luther Martin Luther (1483–1546), the German reformer, theologian and writer, mounted a lifelong struggle against the established Church, greatly influencing Christianity. For the dogmatic canine.

Lyall *See* **Leo**.

Lysander In Shakespeare's *A Midsummer Night's Dream* Lysander is the lover of Hermia, who has been ordered by her father to marry Demetrius, who in turn loves her friend Helena.

M

Maclaren *See* **Bentley**.

Mad Hatter If you've got a crazy but sociable dog, name him after the host of the bizarre tea-party at which Alice finds herself during her adventures in Wonderland in Lewis Carroll's classic children's story.

Mafeking A regimental dog in the Boer War belonging to a detachment under the command of Baden-Powell. Mafeking briefly stopped the crossfire when he wandered out into the middle of the battlefield.

Maida Another of Sir Walter Scott's dogs. *See* **Camp**.

Major Extremely popular, and quite fitting for an old, fuddy-duddy gun dog.

Mandy *See* **Amanda**.

Marmaduke If you have a big, clumsy and lovable Great Dane, then this name, from the famous cartoon strip *Marmaduke*, will suit him down to the ground.

Mars The red planet and Roman god. *See* **Deimos**.

Martha Paul McCartney of Beatles fame immortalized his dog Martha in a song he wrote about her.

Mathe King Richard II's dog. When the king was deposed by Henry of Lancaster, Mathe, without a backward glance, switched his affections to the usurper. For the cur who bites the hand that feeds it.

Matilda Another name of Old German derivation, this one means 'mighty battlemaid'. It became popular in England after the Norman invasion because it was the name of the wife of William the Conqueror. Tillie is a popular short form.

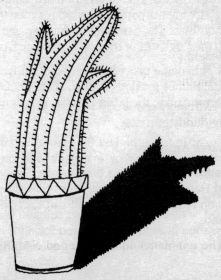

Maximilian Means 'greatest'. Short form is Max. Usually given to dogs of the larger breeds, particularly German Shepherds, Dobermann Pinschers, Great Danes, Newfoundlands and Old English Sheepdogs.

Melba A dog with some vocal ability would be required to fill the shoes of the famous opera singer Dame Nellie Melba.

Melville Name your dog for Herman Melville, author of *Moby Dick*, and you may find that your pet has a taste for fish – with a vengeance.

Merlin The Prince of Enchanters. Son of a damsel seduced by a fiend, baptized and so rescued from the power of Satan. The name of the soothsayer of the King Arthur legend. For the dog with a touch of magic.

Michael This name provides many diminutives that are ideal names for dogs – Mike, Mick, Mickey, Mogga and Spike, the latter two being recent short forms. *See* **Spike**.

Millicent Again from the Old German, this name means 'strong worker' or 'energetic' and can be abbreviated to Millie.

Milton The great seventeenth-century poet and author of *Paradise Lost*, John Milton put religion back into Renaissance thought. A shortened form for a less highbrow canine could be Milt or even Miltie.

Ming Meaning 'bright', this was the name adopted by the founder of the Chinese dynasty of the same name, from whence came the priceless Ming vases. For the decorative-looking dog.

Mr Dog 'A dog with money is addressed as Mr Dog' – Spanish proverb.

Mogga *See* **Michael**.

Mongo This comes from a Greek word meaning 'hoarse' and was the nickname of Peter, Monophysite, Patriarch of Alexandria (*c.* AD 490). A good name for a silent dog who wags its tail instead of barking for joy.

Monroe Perfect for a dazzling dog or captivating canine. Name her for the one and only Marilyn. Alternatively, it's a good name for the fleabag with the *Seven Year Itch*.

Moolah If your dog is consuming a large proportion of your income or cost a lot to purchase, you could call it Moolah – slang for money.

Moomin Perhaps your dog resembles the small, amiable hippo-like animals Tove Jansson created in the *Moomintrolls* rather than a conventional canine. Moomintroll companions include Sniff, Snufkin, Groke, the Snork Maiden and the long-haired Muskrat.

Mopser 'Has anybody seen my Mopser?
– A comely dog is he,
With hair the colour of Charles the Fifth,
And teeth like ships at sea.'

– Walter de la Mare, *The Bandog*

Morgan Full name: Morgan le Fay, fairy sister of King Arthur, *fae* being Old French for 'fairy'. For the dog who is light on its feet.

Muffin This is a cuddly-sounding name loved by children, and it would suit a golden-brown-coloured dog.

Murphy Murphy's law states that if anything can go wrong, it will. If your dog is suitably cynical, then this moniker would be appropriate. Be warned, though, that Murphy is also slang for a potato.

Muskrat *See* **Moomin**.

Muttley For a dog that giggles like Dick Dastardly's double-crossing sidekick in the TV cartoon *Wacky Races*.

N

Nana J.M. Barrie's name for the huge dog in *Peter Pan* who is loving nursemaid to the three Darling children, Wendy, John and Michael.

Natasha After the heroine of Tolstoy's *War and Peace*. A lovely name for a dog of Russian breeding. Other Russian possibilities could be **Nina, Anna** or **Tanya**.

Ned Ned Kelly was a famous Australian bush-ranger. For a dog with a rebellious streak.

Nehru Jawaharlal, the first Prime Minister of India, of great stature and eminence. For the independent dog.

Nell After Nell Gwyn, the beautiful mistress of Charles II.

Nelson There have been many famous Nelsons throughout history, including Babyface Nelson, the American gangster; Viscount Horatio Nelson, the English naval hero, and Nelson Mandela, the President of of the ANC in South Africa.

Nero After the Roman tryant who fiddled while Rome burned. For the dog who watches burglars but doesn't stop them.

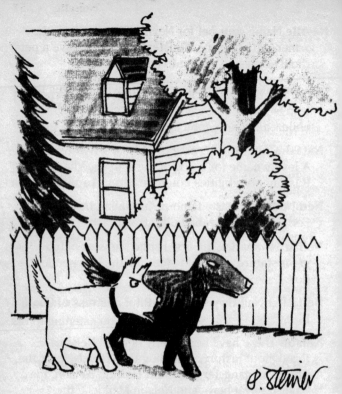

'It's always "Sit", "Stay", "Heel" – never "Think", "Innovate", "Be yourself"'.

Drawing by P. Steiner; © 1990 The New Yorker Magazine, Inc.

Neville Name your pet for Neville Chamberlain, the former British Prime Minister, and you'll have a pet who'll always be willing to appease you.

Newton After Sir Isaac. For the dog who realizes that what goes up must come down. *See* **Diamond**.

Nick Nick Charles, the hero of the Thin Man films. A good name for a bloodhound or other tracking dog.

Nimbus A name that carries more romance than one initially imagines. The *Oxford English Dictionary* describes nimbus as 'a bright cloud, or cloudlike splendour, imagined as investing deities when they appeared on earth'. Does this sound like your dog?

Nina *See* **Natasha**.

Nipper If you think your dog appreciates good music, then name him after the small black-and-white dog who is pictured on RCA record labels listening to his master's voice.

Niven After the late actor David Niven. For a suave and gentlemanly dog.

Nodel See **Reynard**.

Noisette This is a type of rose named for Philippe Noisette, who first introduced it. It is a cross between a common China rose and a musk rose.

Norman It is interesting to note that this name was quite common before the Norman Conquest but died out in England during the Middle Ages. Norm and Normie, the common and affectionate diminutives, are perhaps less severe.

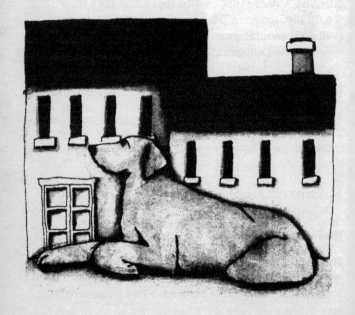

O

Obelix Asterix's partner in adventure and the consumer of great quantities of wild boar. *See* **Asterix**, **Dogmatix**.

Odessa Name your dog for this Russian city, locale of Eisenstein's *Battleship Potemkin*, and you may find her a bit mutinous.

Old Yeller The family dog who contracts rabies and has to be shot in the Hollywood weepie of the same name.

Orson Your pooch will be honoured to be named for Orson Welles, the great actor and film-maker – but remember, Orson was rather portly . . .

Oscar Meaning 'God-spear', Oscar is the name of many famous people: Oscar Hammerstein, Oscar Wilde, Oscar Niemeyer and the film industry awards – the Oscars. Also suitable for a pair of total opposites, like Oscar and **Felix** in *The Odd Couple*.

P

Pablo *See* **Picasso**.

Paddington The only name for a dog from deepest, darkest Peru, found in a train station with a sign saying 'Please look after this dog' around its neck. Must have a fondness for marmalade.

Pal The first star of the Lassie films was, in fact, a laddie called Pal who lived a life of luxury during his film career. He was retired to a ranch after five years of making films, where he lived to the age of nineteen.

Pandy In Dodie Smith's *101 Dalmatians* Pandy is the smallest and youngest of the ill-fated litter of pups that falls into Cruella de Ville's evil hands.

Pasha An attractive name, which is the title in Turkey of officers of high rank in military or civic positions. For the dignified dog.

Pavlov The perfect name for the dog whose breed is noted for its excessive drooling or always knows when it's time for dinner.

Pavlova For a dog who is light on its toes or who likes sweet things.

Pegasus The winged horse on whose back Bellerophon rode against the mythical monster the Chimera. Would suit a dog with stature, like a Great Dane or a Dobermann.

Penn William Penn, Quaker leader or Sean Penn, 'Brat Pack' member. For dogs with a range of temperament.

Percy *See* **Dudley**.

Perdy Devoted partner to **Pongo** and mother of his pups in *101 Dalmations*.

Peri A fairy-like or elfin being in Persian mythology.

Perites Alexander the Great's favourite canine was the last of an illustrious breed of dog that could slay a lion in a matter of minutes. An ideal name for a guard dog.

Peter Peter the Great established Russia as northern Europe's leading military power. If, much to your relief, your hound is not in the least bit warlike, then name him after St Peter, who was devoted to Jesus.

Petie The dog from *The Little Rascals*. Many a pup's a little rascal – here's a name for your little one.

Phobos *See* **Deimos**.

Picasso For the dog who has his Blue Periods but also his Pink Periods, and, if your canine resembles a cube, all the better.

Pickles The terrier shopkeeper in Beatrix Potter's *Ginger and Pickles*. Ginger is a yellow cat.

Pickwick If your dog loves to rove around, taking a great interest in everything he sees, name him after Charles Dickens's humorous traveller.

Pinscher A Dobermann, of course.

Pip The perfect name for a puppy, if you have Great Expectations for him. In Dickens's novel Pip is an orphan, befriended by Magwitch, an escaped convict, who becomes his benefactor.

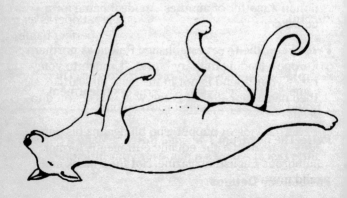

Pluto A very popular name for black dogs. In mythology Pluto was god of his own dark realm, the entrance to which was guarded by a huge three-headed dog, Cerberus. Also the name of a popular Walt Disney dog.

Pongo In *101 Dalmatians* by Dodie Smith, Pongo is the father of the stolen litter of puppies. *See* **Perdy**.

Prince There's a Prince for almost every breed – Prince of Darkness (Satan); Prince of Wales (Charles); Prince of Humbug (Phineas T. Barnum, the circus owner); Prince of Destruction (Timur the Lame, the Mongol conqueror renowned for his cruelty); Prince of Artists (Albrecht Dürer, the great German artist). And the list goes on. *See* **Goldie**.

Princess *See* **Duchess**.

Puccini The Italian composer of such great operas as *Madame Butterfly* and *La Bohème*. The perfect name for the favourite pet of a musical family.

Pumpkin For a beast acquired at Hallow'en. The name is used by some as a term of endearment. Could denote an orange-brown colour.

Punch That violent puppet who bludgeons his wife Judy to death. Or the equally outrageous former humorous English magazine. Not for a meek and mild mutt.

Q

Queenie *See* **Duchess**.

Quincy If your dog has an ear for music, why not name him after Quincy Jones, famous record producer for Michael Jackson, Tina Turner, and Liza Minnelli, to name a few.

R

Raffles Sir Thomas Stamford Bingley Raffles (1781–1826), British founder of Singapore. Also the gentleman burglar and cricketer in novels by E.W. Hornung. An apt name for a risk-taker, with connotations of lottery and gambling, derived from a game of chance of that name.

Ralph This means 'counsel-wolf', and is both an Old Norse and an Anglo-Saxon name. It's the sort of name that suits the feistier, less sensitive breeds of dog.

Ramekin Or Ramequin. Sounds like a fabulous fictional name. Use it for that fairy-tale dog, though remember that, literally, it applies to something small. Wonderful for a Bichon Frise.

Randolph This can be abbreviated to Randy, a popular name in America for audacious mutts. It is more popular in England in its longer form, being a family name of the Marlboroughs.

Rasputin The Russian monk and mystic, known for his drunkenness, sexual excess and nepotism. An enigmatic, exotic name, but use it cautiously, as it may have arcane powers.

Remus *See* **Romulus**.

Reynard The beast-epic poem *Roman de Renart*, of
the fourteenth century, is a satire on the state of
Germany in the Middle Ages, with the church
represented by Reynard the fox, the baronial classes
represented by the wolf **Isengrin** and royalty by
Nodel the lion.

Riley There are times when a person feels that his dog
has a more comfortable and jolly life than he does –
in fact, 'a life of Riley'. A good name for a much-
loved family pet.

Rin Tin Tin Canine hero of film fame. What dog
wouldn't be flattered to be named after one of the
world's great movie stars?

Rocky After the series of Sylvester Stallone films about
an Italian American boxer, an obvious name for a
Boxer dog.

Roger Yet another war-derived name, this one
comes from Anglo-Saxon words meaning 'fame'
and 'spear', and was a very popular name from the
time of the Domesday Book until the sixteenth
century.

Roller *See* **Bentley**.

Romulus One of the twin sons of Mars and Rhea
   Silvia, who were suckled by a she-wolf after their
   mother was slain. They began building Rome but
   argued, and Romulus killed his brother **Remus**.
   Perfect for canine sibling rivals.

Rory With clearly rolled r's, this is a grand name for a
   dog of an Irish or a Scottish breed.

Rose As Shakespeare put it in *Romeo and Juliet*:

> What's in a name? That which we call a rose
> By any other name would smell as sweet.

Rover A bit common. Do not expect this pooch to be
   home in time for dinner. A wandering cur with a
   definite wild streak, a bit of a cad and highly
   unreliable.

Rubens Sir Peter Paul, the prolific Flemish painter,
   famous for his fleshy women. A wonderful name for
   the female with a 'Renaissance' figure who is
   colourful, exotic and sensual, like the paintings.

Ruby In the nineteenth century, jewel names became
   popular, and the name Ruby was among them. The
   first recorded use of the name is in 'John Peel', the
   old English hunting song, in which one of the
   hounds is called Ruby.

Rudolph Only to be used if the mutt comes into your life at Christmas, or if he really does have a red nose, like the famed reindeer.

Rufus This name is of Latin derivation, meaning 'red' or 'reddish'. It has been bestowed as a nickname upon many famous people, including William II of England in reference to his ruddy complexion.

Rugby This game started in the public schools of England but its combination of rough-and-tumble and skill soon made it popular throughout many different clubs and world-wide. A good name for an exuberant dog who loves to chase and roll in the mud.

Russell For a Jack Russell Terrier.

Rusty When the colour of your dog is a pretty indiscriminate mix of red and brown, then no other name will do but Rusty.

S

Sacha, Sasha An elegant name for male or female, Sacha is short for Alexander. Suitable for a Borzoi or an Afghan hound.

Sally This name is suitable for a small female dog with a twinkle in her eye and a bounce to her step but will not do for a larger dog with family responsibilities.

Salome You will know at once whether your bitch is a Salome, a sinuous, hypnotic name. It would suit a Greyhound or any slender female with the right qualities.

Samson Dogs are intuitive, and the name will suggest to him all your expectations. This is not suitable for a breed that is traditionally close-shorn.

Sandy If it is made clear that the dog's name is Alexander, you may suffer no embarrassment; after all, the kids chose it. It should bear some relation to the dog's colouring.

Sarah For Sarah Bernhardt, the French tragedienne who played both male and female roles and who came to be known as the Divine Sarah.

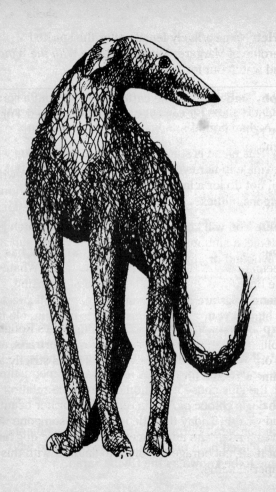

Scarlett Name a lively female after the spirited heroine of Margaret Mitchell's *Gone With the Wind* – and watch out for trouble!

Scooby Doo The lovable cartoon dog without a scrap of courage that loves to eat when he's scared. For the type of dog who would lead burglars to the family silver.

Scrappy Doo The young nephew of Scooby Doo who has too much bravado. Faces dangerous situations with a war cry of 'Puppy Power!' A good name for a fearless pup.

Shane The right name for an Irish Setter, but it has been known as the name for a Dachshund. Whatever the breed, you'll never be ashamed of choosing Shane.

Sharp This was the name of Queen Victoria's Rough Collie. He can be seen in several royal portraits, and in one he is seated by the throne. This is strictly a name for regal breeds.

Sheba The Queen of Arabia renowned for her beauty and wealth. Today the title is used for someone who gives herself airs and graces. If your exotic dog has got it all, encourage the bitch to flaunt it with this imperial name.

Siegfried This name, associated more often these days with the popular TV show *All Creatures Great and Small* than with grand opera, could be used for most dogs, although it would be more common among those of German extraction. Highly recommended.

Sirius Sirius is not often used as a dog's name, but it should be, because Sirius is the Dog Star and the brightest in the night sky.

Skip/Skippy Only for a very bouncy dog, after Australia's most famous bush kangaroo, star of the *Skippy* TV series.

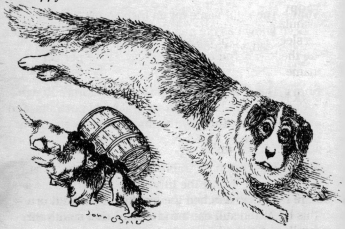

Drawing by John O'Brien; © 1990 The New Yorker Magazine, Inc.

Skipper A very jolly name, though sea dogs are rare.
There are two indications: he may be the leader of
the litter or just a lively little chap.

Sly Sylvester 'Sly' Stallone. For the very muscular
breeds. Or use it more literally if he's crafty or
devious.

Smuts *See* **Sooty**.

Snap So long as he is kept on a leash there should be
no trouble.

Sniff *See* **Moomin**.

Snoopy The lovable beagle created by Charles M.
Schulz in the *Peanuts* comic strip. If your dog tends
to sleep on top of his kennel or pretends to
be the Red Baron or Joe Cool, this is the perfect
name.

Snork Maiden *See* **Moomin**.

Snowball, Snowflake *See* **Sooty**.

Snufkin *See* **Moomin**.

Soda *See* **Whisky**.

Softie If you've searched the length and breadth of
this book and still can't find a name that suits your
family pet, then this is a last resort.

Sooty Together with Snowflake, Smuts and Snowball, this name either states the obvious or is used in jest – for example, naming a black kitten Snowflake.

Spam The much maligned luncheon meat. A good, fun name for a mutt of indefinable breeding.

Spike A name growing in popularity. It calls to mind Spike Milligan, the famous Goon, an animal lover and activist. You will know a Spike when you see one.

Spitz Another character from Jack London's *Call of the Wild*, the classic tale of rivalry and survival of the fittest in a husky pack in the inhospitable North. Spitz is the pack leader whose place Buck usurps.

Sport An affectionate nickname, appropriate for a gamester.

Spot Not a name for the discerning, however obvious the spot may be, although fans of Eric Hill's well-loved children's book and television character may feel differently. It would probably do very well for a mongrel with a spot, owned by a family with children.

Sprat Perfect for the lean or fussy hound who may or may not be partnered with a female who can eat no lean meat.

Stanley Kubrick, legendary American film director responsible for such films as *Lolita, A Clockwork Orange* and, more recently, *Full Metal Jacket*. A name for only a very unusual and extraordinary dog.

Star If your dog moves like a meteor, fights like **Mars** and eats like a black hole, yet is the light of your life, perhaps this is just the name.

Stella Stella is Latin for 'star' and was first used as a name by Sir Philip Sidney. His collection of sonnets and songs named *Astrophel and Stella* (*c.* 1582) was written for Lady Penelope Devereux, whom he was wooing.

Sullivan *See* **Gilbert**.

Sultan This is a noble, kingly name; one envisages a large, sleek creature, perfectly trained.

Susie Like Sally, this name is without distinction, despite the suggestion of amiability and sunshine. Would be quite suitable for a small unpretentious Cairn.

Swift After the English satirist Jonathan Swift. Also rapid or fast, for the speedy breeds such as Greyhounds and Whippets.

T

Taff/Taffy A familiar form of address or nickname for a Welshman, derived from the Welsh pronunciation of Davy or David. Taffy can mean blarney, sweet-talking or coarse flattery.

Taggy, Talgert Derived from **Agnes**, as is **Annis**. Very pleasing names for short and friendly breeds.

Talbot The Talbot hound is a now-extinct breed of hound used for tracking in the sixteenth century, a large pale-coloured dog with long, hanging ears and great powers of smell. Chaucer used this as a dog's name.

Tango The code word to represent the letter 'T', a seductive Argentine ballroom dance or its music. This is a versatile name.

Tanya *See* **Natasha**.

Tarquin When Tarquinius Sextus raped Lucretia, the Tarquins were expelled from Rome and the Republic set up in their place. Be warned: your pooch could become a blackguardly cur under the influence of this name.

Tennessee In the prologue to *Camino Real* American
playwright Tennessee Williams wrote, 'It is a terrible
thing for an old woman to outlive her dogs.' Still, a
good name for the dog with dramatic flair.

Thisbe This amusing, gay little name brings to mind
the workmen's play in *A Midsummer Night's Dream*.
It was also the name of Marie Antionette's toy
spaniel, given to her by way of apology by Louis XVI
(who killed her own little dog in a fit of rage).

Tillie *See* **Matilda**.

Tiny Another name used best ironically.

Titus Titus (*c.* AD 39–81) was a Roman emperor who
put an end to treason trials and drove out informers.
Almost all hostilities ceased during his reign. For a
dog who longs for the peaceful life.

Toby From the Hebrew 'Tobias', this means 'the Lord
is good'. **Punch**'s dog (in Punch and Judy) bears the
name.

Tolstoy After Leo, author of *War and Peace* – an
appropriate description of life in many households.

Tosca An opera by Puccini. Beware of an inclination
towards the tragic. Masculine is **Tosco**, but the
feminine sounds better.

Toto Dorothy's beloved little dog in *The Wizard of Oz*.

Towser A name first used in the seventeenth century for a large dog, particularly those used to bait bears or bulls. Only for those owners who are fond of blood sports.

Trixie This is the short form of **Beatrice** and quite a common name for dainty little dogs.

Trotsky Leon Trotsky, Stalin's nemesis, exiled from Russia in 1929 and assassinated in Mexico in 1940. For a Chihuahua or any dog who likes a good run in the morning.

Truffe Childhood pet of Alexandre Dumas, author of *The Three Musketeers*. The dog was obviously of massive proportions, as Dumas remembered riding on its back.

Truffles For the dog who's always nosing around.

Trumper Trumpery is fraud, imposture or trickery. A good name for the mutt who continually hoodwinks you.

Trusty Perhaps after the bloodhound in Walt Disney's *Lady and the Tramp*, but this is a risky name to give a young dog unless you are happy with irony.

V

Valentine This would be a perfect name for a gift of love, after St Valentine's Day, 14 February, the day of lovers, which is named for a Christian martyred in Rome (*c.* 270).

Verne For Jules Verne, the great science-fiction writer. For the dog who sometimes makes you wish you could send him to the moon.

Vespucci (Spelled Vespoochi??) After Amerigo Vespucci, the Italian navigator.

Victor This name needs no explanation, having been adopted into English directly from the Latin. It would suit those breeds known for their ability to win the fight – Rottweilers and Bull Terriers come quickly to mind.

Vigi Vigi was a large, shaggy iron-grey hound from Gaelic legend that was adopted by Olaf I, King of the Vikings, for his cleverness and speed.

Vincent Van Gogh (1853–1890). A Dutch painter much influenced by Impressionism. His work has recently sold for record prices, but his image in the popular mind is much influenced by his mental instability. Appropriate for a dog with one ear.

Virgil Roman poet (70–19 BC). Virgil's *Georgics* (36–29 BC) is a four-volume agricultural treatise, written with characteristic pathos and love, reporting careful observation of animals and nature. *See* **George**.

Viva A shout or exclamation from the Italian, meaning 'Long live!' A great, exuberant name to call out loud.

Vixen This name has a great ring to it. It is the name for a female fox or traditionally means a shrewish or quarrelsome woman. For the fiery redhead.

Vladimir Vladimir I (956–1015) was a Ukrainian-Scandinavian saint. Once an unruly Viking, he converted to Christianity and married, then brought his religion to his subjects. For the born-again mutt.

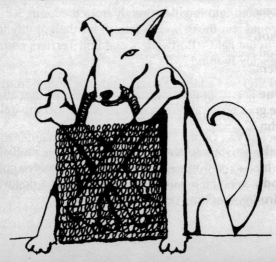

W

Waldo A name that recalls that old scamp in *Under Milk Wood* by Dylan Thomas. The name originates from the Old English Waltheof, a compound of 'power', 'rule' and, unfortunately, 'thief'.

Wamba In Sir Walter Scott's *Ivanhoe* (1820), the jester of Cedric the Saxon. For the dog whose antics make you laugh and whose devotion warms your heart.

Washington Good name for a dog of American descent, even though this name originates from the ancient English village Wassa and actually means 'home of the people of Wassa'.

Watson Dr Watson, Sherlock **Holmes**'s partner. A good name for a smart dog who's always overshadowed by true genius.

Wayne If your dog's a real son of a gun, call him after the greatest of all Western heroes, the incomparable John Wayne.

Whisky This would make a good name for a Scottish- or Irish-bred dog, especially one with a golden coat. **Soda** could be a pair name or would suit a dog with a frothy, sparkling personality.

Wilbur Another name from the Old German, this one means 'will' and 'defence'. Wilbur was the name of one of the Wright brothers, the aviation pioneers.

William Will is the obvious diminutive if your dog is a little prince.

Wimbledon Celebrate the tradition of the famous grass courts tournament if your dog is white or loves to chase a ball.

Windsor Popular with British royalty, the Corgi was introduced to Queen Elizabeth II by her father when he was Duke of York. Rozavel Golden Eagle, better known as Dookie, was their first dog.

Winston This name derives from a hamlet in Gloucestershire of the same name. It is also associated with British Prime Minister Sir Winston Churchill. His resemblance to little babies and Bulldogs has resulted in many small creatures bearing the name.

Wodehouse Pelham Grenville Wodehouse (1881–1975) wrote over 120 volumes and created well-loved characters including **Jeeves**, the wise and resourceful valet, and his amiable but vacuous employer, Bertie **Wooster**.

Wolf *See* **Goldie**.

Woodhouse The English dog trainer Barbara Woodhouse is claimed in *The Guinness Book of Records* to have been the most successful trainer of dogs. A good name for those dogs who need constant reminders of obedience.

Woodruff A woodland herb found in Britain and Europe; it has small white flowers and strongly scented leaves. For those with a strong doggy smell.

Wooster *See* **Jeeves**, **Wodehouse**.

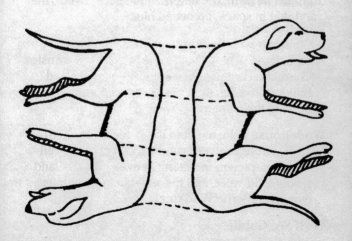

Y

Yahoo A brute with human form and rough and uncouth manner, from Swift's *Gulliver's Travels*.

Yogi For Yogi Bear, the bumbling bruin of Jellystone Park. *See* **Boo Boo.**

Yorick For the jester who's always digging up bones.

Yuppie For the Young Urban Pet with the most up-to-date accessories. For your yuppie puppie.

Yuri Yuri Gagarin, the first man in space. **Laika**, the first dog in space, preceded him.

Z

Zappa Frank Zappa, avant-garde musician. Zappa named his children Dweezil and Moon Unit, so don't hesitate to name your dog for him – he won't be offended.

Zara Marasquin de Zara is a renowned liqueur made at Zara, a Dalmatian village situated on the Adriatic. The liqueur is much used in pastry and confectionery. Sounds like a dog's name.

Zebedee If your dog's always bouncing around, call him after the springy character in the children's TV series *The Magic Roundabout*.

Zeppo One of the Marx Brothers. *See* **Groucho**.

Zeste From French for 'peel'; it means something which gives relish or flavour. An appropriate name for an important addition to the family, particularly one with strong inclinations and gusto.

Zeta The sixth letter of the Greek alphabet, and it has a great sound to it. This name could be useful if the number six is significant. Perhaps you could call your sixth dog this.

Ziegfeld Flo Ziegfeld, theatrical producer. If every walk with your pooch requires elaborate preparation.

Zingano/Zingaro This name means 'gypsy' in Italian and is a suitable name for a pooch with a wanderlust.

Zip A speedy dog who sets the pace for the morning jog.

Zoe This is the Greek version of the name Eve, meaning 'life'. It was a popular name in the Roman Empire, then in England after about 1850 and, most recently, in the United States.

Zoilus Or, in Greek, Zoilos. He was a shrewd, witty and harsh critic of Homer, Plato and Isocrates. He was nicknamed 'Homer's scourge' for his assault on the *Odyssey*.

Zorba Can your dog dance? Then name him after the hero of the movie *Zorba the Greek*.

MORE POCKET PENGUINS

published or forthcoming